LOSE WEIGHT FAST WITHOUT DIETING

(SAY NO TO DIETS)

LEONARDO DOMÍNGUEZ

Lose weight without a dieting

1st Edition 2020

Direction Leonardo Dominguez

Cover design

Rodchenko

Diagramming

Farell Luizaga

Translate

Victor_estevez

ACKNOWLEDGMENT

I give thanks to many people for having encouraged me to write this book and to all who have given their grain of sand with a great advice.

This book is dedicated to my family, especially my mother and father. I also thank my nutritionist for supporting me in doing this project when I mentioned it.

And to you for buying this book. THANK YOU.

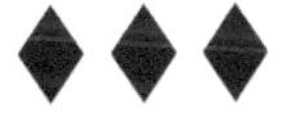

CONTENT

CHAPTER 1 8

CHAPTER II 12

MY 7 TIPS TO LOSE WEIGHT 12

CHAPTER III 16

¿ LOSE WEIGHT? 16

DON´T DO MORE DIETS 16

CHAPTER IV 20

FLEXIBLE FEEDING' 20

CHAPTER V 24

3 TIPS TO START WITH FLEXIBLE FOOD 24

CHAPTER VI 26

FLEXIBLE FEEDING 26

CHAPTER VII 30

FOODS YOU SHOULD BUY TO LOSE WEIGHT 30

(FLEXIBLE) 30

CHAPTER VIII 36

HEALTHY NUTRITION 36

CHAPTER IX 40

INTERMITTENT FASTING 40

THIS IS GOLD! 40

CHAPTER X 44

FROM OBESE TO HAVING A RIPPED ABDOMEN 44

CHAPTER XI 46

5 LIES OF THE FITNESS 46

CHAPTER XII 48

CARDIO TO LOSE WEIGHT 48

WEIGHTS ARE BETTER THAN CARDIO 54

(MEN AND WOMEN) 54

CHAPTER XIII 58

REDUCE WAIST AND ABDOMEN FAT 58

CHAPTER XIV 62

CALORIC DEFICIT 62

CHAPTER XV 64

COUNTING, ESTIMATING MACROS IS IMPORTANT FOR WEIGHT LOSS 64

MACROS AND CUSTOMIZATION TO LOSE WEIGHT IN MYFITNESSPAL 70

CHAPTER XVI 74

CALORIE CYCLE PER WEEK. 74

CHAPTER XVII 78

LOSE FAT AND NOT MUSCLE 78

CHAPTER XVIII 80

YOU DON'T LOSE WEIGHT? 80

(ACCELERATE YOUR METABOLISM) 80

CHAPTER XIXSUPPLEMENTS? 82

(HERBALIFE, VIVRI, OMNILIFE, DETOX,) 82

CHAPTER XX 86

I AM ENDOMORPH AND MESOMORPH HOW SHOULD I LOSE WEIGHT? 86

CHAPTER XXI 88

CARBOHYDRATES ARE YOUR ALLIES 88

CHAPTER XXII 90

YOUR SOCIAL LIFE IS MORE IMPORTANT DO NOT RESTRICT OR LIMIT YOURSELF!
....90

CHAPTER XXIII 94

PROBLEMS (STRESS, CELLULITE, EXCESS SKIN AND DISEASES)..................94

CHAPTER XXIV 96

IF YOU WANT TO CHANGE THINGS, DON'T ALWAYS DO THE SAME 96

CHAPTER XXV 98

MOTIVATION (LIVE YOUR LIFE BE HAPPY!) 98

CHAPTER XXVI...100

15 QUESTIONS ABOUT LOSING WEIGHT (UNISEX) 100

CONCLUSION 103

BEFORE YOU GO 104

CHAPTER 1

Introduction

"Insanity is doing the same thing over and over again, but expecting different results."

- Albert Einstein

After having spent more than 2 years without losing weight in diets, programs, having bought products and pills to lose weight and approximately after having gone through an obsession period that I do not recommend to anyone, I decided to start applying what I learned with the truth and stop fooling around with diets and other trends such as products, belts, pills and restrictions that all I did was make things worse.

When you are a young you start worrying about your weight or your physical appearance and when you start wanting to be thin, with a good body you look for and absorb information and many lies about the reality of losing weight.

My earlier days

- Going to the institute and try to eat as little as possible to follow the diet.

- Going out of class and eating whatever there was for lunch, having seconds and ice cream, and then feeling bad for having eaten all that food.

- I felt bad for not following the instructions of the weight loss plan. If I went out with friends or with my brothers that afternoon, I drank a lot of soda and a bag of potato chips, Doritos, Pringles or candy. I won´t tell you that I ate in the afternoon and when dinner arrived.

I would send everything to hell when I couldn't resist, and could not keep up with the diet organized by the coach. I started with other diets of limitations in absolutely everything, no starches, no carbohydrates, all gluten free and super "healthy" I spent my savings on meats and products that were 'necessary' for my 'diet' apart from that, I used creams and pills that They said and I thought worked.

I felt with low energy (obviously because of the abrupt lack of reducing carbohydrates), and I kept gaining fat. As I was doing everything perfect to the diet plan! I ate lots of fruits, meats and vegetables, lots of products and only drank water. Obviously, since you are not used to it, you end up giving up that lifestyle, you end up feeling guilty and resorting to bingeing…

I discovered a meal plan in which going out to dinner with friends was fun and it was guilty free for food, traveling, eating out with acquaintances and friends I was happy to discover new foods, exercise only 20 to 30 minutes with weights and cardio daily had a purpose and was not simply a way to 'lose weight' nor did I feel guilty for not training every day a week cardio.

I learned a lifestyle of eating everything and basing my diet on what I like and my body needs such as macronutrients (proteins, carbohydrates, healthy fats), I have learned that food and social life are for living and enjoying.

There is no trick, diets, or miraculous recipes for losing weight.
What do exist are feeding systems or medium or long term systems.

To lose weight you need to look for a system that will take you where you want to go.
I have studied this subject very well and I can firmly say that there are systems or "diets" that do not require effort or restrictions.

To lose weight, I recommend reading this book, studying it, taking it with you and creating a habit in your reading. In which I tell you the methods I use and the best system to lose weight. This method worked for me to have the body I longed to have.

Everything is achieved with effort, dedication and adherence.

Recommend this book to your loved ones and friends who need them,
They will thank you very much.

Greetings, and God bless you!

Chapter II
MY 7 TIPS TO LOSE WEIGHT

1. Stop eating - Under no circumstances make abrupt changes in the calories you consume!
Your change of diet has to be gradual, "follow the law of inertia."

If you suddenly stop consuming carbohydrates, chances are that you lower your intake and end up stalling.

2. Calorie Deficit - It is to reduce your calories that you consume or need your body. Your body needs an estimate of calories, it is not relative since each person is different, but there is an estimate of what is spent.

By making a deficit means that --- if you consume 3000 calories, then you lower 500 calories to your daily intake, your body will get used to the new caloric intake, then you will lose weight.
Do not forget to lower gradually and with good intake of macronutrients, not suddenly.
ROME WASN´T BUILT IN A DAY

3. Flexible feeding- I don't consider it a diet because it is a diet system without having to restrict you from any food.

This system allows you not to feel on a diet, it does not imply sacrifice or food restrictions.
I remember I was on diets to maintain my body, many of them involve food restrictions, and obviously I ended up giving up because I couldn't stand that kind of diet with many restrictions.

4. Choose your best plan or system in the medium or long term - You must choose a food system that does not represent sacrifice, otherwise you will end up giving up!

 Applies to all existing diets, miracle recipes or detoxifications, all work in the medium or long term. You have the decision to choose a system - a system that you like! But that you do it in medium or long term.

5. To progress you have to count what you do (count, estimate macronutrients).
In life everything is a number, to be successful you have to learn to count numbers, the money you receive, mathematical operations or daily life.

If you don't count what you give or what you receive in your daily life, whether in life or in food, you are lost!

If it is measurable it can be improved

I don't mean to count your calories and everything you eat, but to "estimate." It is better to count than not to count because if you don't, you will not know what you have or what you consume.

6. Burn fat (Intermittent fasting) - Intermittent fasting is a great challenge to burn fat.

It is not a recipe or magical wand, "it is only a help", fasting is to reduce your caloric intake, "eat what you want, just eat when you are hungry" is called flexibility.
In this book I will talk more deeply about intermittent fasting.

7. 65% and 35% - Food is 65% of the results and training routines only affect your results by 35%.

If you want to burn a good cardio routine fast and whether a man or a woman is good, to start losing calories. Weights burn more calories than cardio.

Conclusion --- Don't be scared I'll take you step by step to the body of your dreams. Keep reading and you will be able to go deeper into each specific topic.

Chapter III
¿ LOSE WEIGHT?
DON´T DO MORE DIETS

One day my friend told me he couldn't lose weight and asked for help, this is the conversation:

Q: "Hello friend, I can't lose weight. In what am I failing?"
A: "What do you eat my friend?"
P: "A light meal, for breakfast 3 buns with avocado and a tamale, for lunch a plate of lentils with tamarind juice, dinner only a quarter of a chicken with rice, sauce and soda"
A: "lower your caloric intake"
Q: "but what? If I'm eating healthy - tamarind, tamale, avocado, aren't they good and can I eat a lot of those?
A: not because they are nutritious in healthy fat means that you can eat a great amount, but what is necessary, in small portions.

It makes no sense to be on a diet and make your life difficult with many food restrictions.
Can't you lose weight? Or have you not been able to lower your body fat? These are 3 reasons why you don't lose weight.

1. Low carbohydrates --- It is essential that you do not last long on a low carb diet.
 If you lower your carb intake abruptly then you will have little energy in your day. What you need is to adapt and gradually lower your carbohydrate intake until your body gets used to it and you can get to eat in a day low amount of carbohydrates.

Many people think that they eat lightly or naturally, but it is confusing to eat "light" with what is nutritious to your body.

2. Nutritious and less nutritious foods --- There are no good or bad foods but only nutritious ones and those that contribute little. Our diet has to be in 65% of foods that provide us with nutrients. Many people think that foods in quotes called "Good" can eat that food as much as they want.
For this reason, you still do not lose weight, for the reason that you are confused in the foods that you think provide value or not.

COUNT — that's why it's good to count the calories and nutrients in each food to make progress on the caloric intake you consume every day.

I recommend **MyFitnessPal**, the fastest and easiest to use calorie counter. It is available on Android, IOS.

Does any diet works?

The true success of a slimming treatment or a diet lies in the possibility of achieving a healthy weight, but, above all, of maintaining such a healthy weight over time as indicated by scientists and thousands of nutrition professionals.

The diets that are in sight are "effective or miraculous" because they allow you to lose a lot of weight in a short time because they include strict, limiting resources without flexibility and therefore, unsustainable over time, that is, they do not generate adherence. There is the rebound effect as demonstrated by research published in the journal Obesity, and therefore, it is impossible to maintain the lost weight which demonstrates the lack of success of the treatment chosen to lose weight.

All diets are good, but if you do not have persistence or your diet has no options to enjoy and you restrict yourself too much you will end up failing, wasting a lot of time and feeling guilty of not achieving your goals.

Chapter IV
Flexible feeding'

The basis for having a muscular body or body defined the diet you want to start has to be sustainable or something that you can carry out without giving up at two or three weeks. "Do not do diets because is trending."

The flexible meal or the so-called flexible diet is a diet without carbohydrate restrictions or fat restrictions. This diet is one of the ones I use the most and it has worked with the people I have given them a coach.

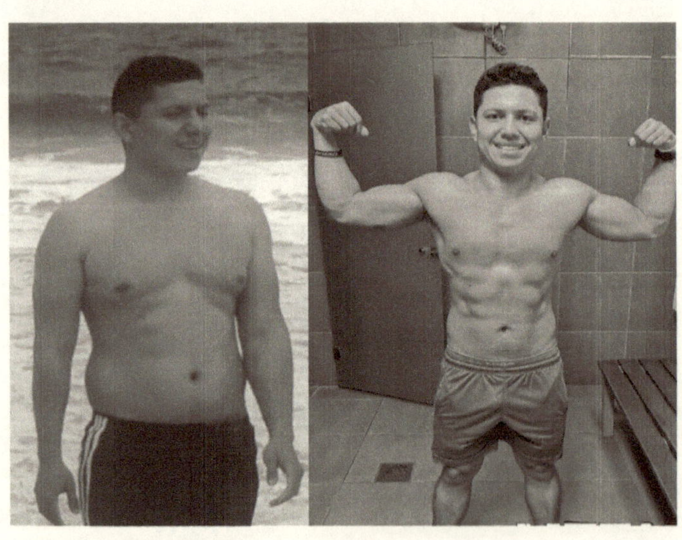

A person who has greatly reduced body fat and has marked his body in just 2 months or 11 weeks.

Don't forget that you have to see losing weight as "a way of life." Never settle; my recommendation is that when you lose weight do not settle and continue living with that lifestyle or the body of dreams you want.

Start with flexible feeding

Flexible feeding is about creating a new way to lose weight without food restrictions, without restrictions on eating what you like once a week, without limitations of eating popcorn or whatever you like.

Nor is it about eating pizzas every day or eating Pancake in the morning or fried chicken. This is a way of eating without having to refuse any event you are invited to, refuse to eat at night with your partner, refuse to eat at family dinners, refuse to eat carbohydrates.
The reason why many people fail in diets with restrictions, **the reason is because the more you restrict yourself --- the more you want it or the more you crave it.**
If you forbid more you will fail.

FLEXIBILITY

You can start with flexible feeding with this tip:

1. 75% and 25% --- The rule is to consume 75% nutritious foods and 25% foods that are not nutritious, but if you can eat foods that make you happy or eat 25% foods without restricting yourself. How to eat popcorn, donuts, French fries, dinner invitations, birthdays, etc.

If you protect yourself from consuming 75% and 25%, believe me it works and you will live happier without any hassle for refusing fun.

Later we will see more detailed about flexible feeding…

Chapter V
3 TIPS TO START WITH FLEXIBLE FOOD

I will share 3 essential points to start with flexible feeding:

1. 75 and 25% --- As I said in the previous chapter 75% healthy foods such as vegetables, vitamins, fruits, cereals, fibers and proteins and 25% to add a taste to life and have no restriction, such as foods that more you like or meals to enjoy with our friends or family. 25% is necessary so that you do not feel restricted and do not leave the plan. It is not necessary to make that percentage necessarily, it can be 80% and 20% or less or more flexible, my advice is so that you do not give up and think you can restrict food.

2. Perseverance — the results appear after 5 weeks, hence everything is in progress. Do not expect to see results in 3, 7, 10 days.

3. Count Nutrients and square them --- (Proteins, carbohydrates and fats) you just have to count what you consume and it should be appropriate for your body.

Later you will see the correct way to count macronutrients.

4. Estimate macros — Estimating what you eat, you can eat whatever you want by calculating what you consumed and what you should no longer consume if you passed the fat or carbohydrate limit. (Estimate macros with **MyFitnessPal or Calorie counter from Android o IOS)**

I show you this kind of diet because it is one of the ones I like the most without having to deprive myself of eating the foods that I love.

The most effective diet is the diet that you can follow the most, that is the diet that best suits your person, the diet that you do not give up and do not refuse to go out and have fun with your social life. **Do not forget that if you want to accelerate the results you should start exercising, any type of exercise is of strength, with your body or sport is valid, that will cause you to burn calories and fat.**

Chapter VI
Flexible feeding

I hope you have not confused that flexible food allows you to eat more than 2,500 calories or more than 3,500 calories, nor is it about eating hamburgers and fried chicken every day but about being flexible in events or situations where you cannot restrict yourself. Flexible feeding is about feeding you with 75% of nutritious foods that provide few calories and 25% foods that are not nutritious, but this is good for not feeling guilty and limited.

Foods to lose weight or be in caloric deficit

1. Strawberry --- When you are in definition or in weight loss, strawberries provide only 9 grams of carbohydrates, and 2 grams of fiber. You can eat a good amount of strawberries in a short time and it will leave you satiated.

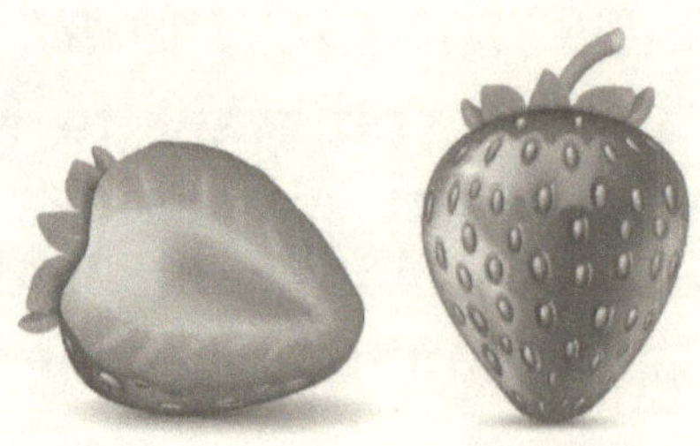

2. Beans --- It contains a small amount of carbohydrates, when you try to lose weight you need to be a little low in carbohydrates, and it only has 1 gram of fat.

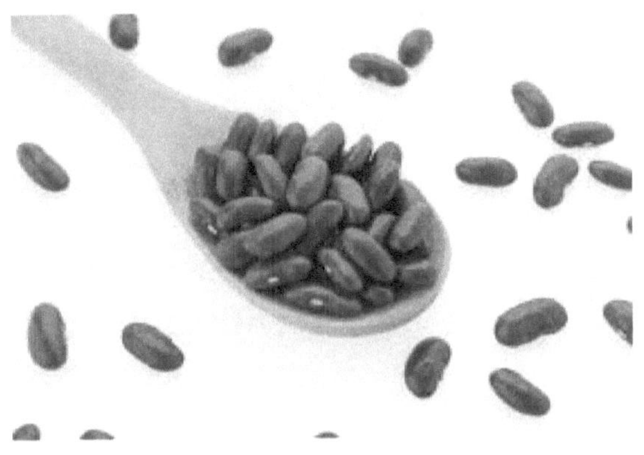

3. Vegetables --- All green food is surprisingly good. A bag of asparagus, lettuce, broccoli or some green food can only give you 15 carbohydrates. To flavor the vegetables, add seasonings.

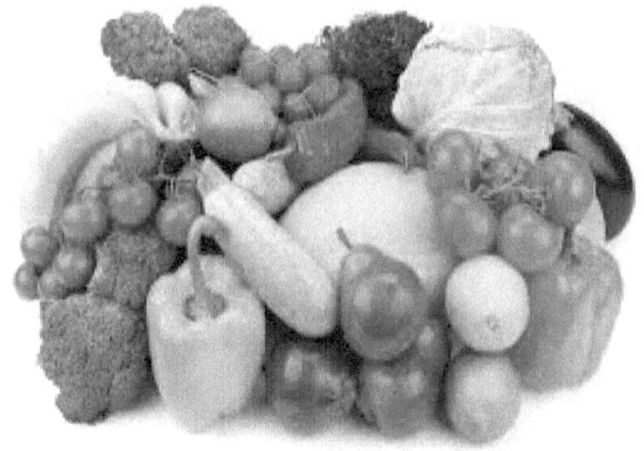

4. Chia --- 40 grams of Chia will help you quench your appetite and help you control some cravings. It contains only 25 gr of carbohydrates.

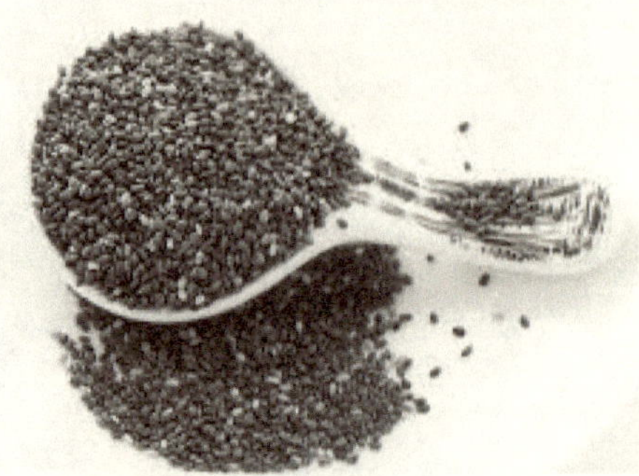

5. Egg whites --- Protein is great for gaining muscle and you have a lot to eat with only 100 gr of egg whites.

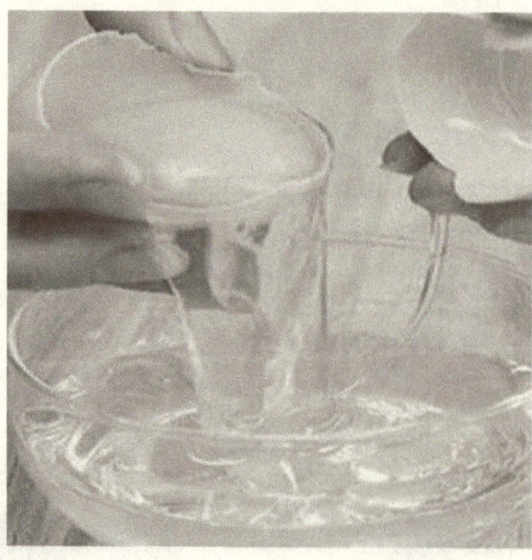

6. Water --- Many times you think you are hungry, but what you have is thirst. If you like soda, I recommend Zero Sugar soda.

7. Intermittent fasting --- It is not mandatory, but it has great power to lose weight. It is about eating only 2 meals a day; at lunch and dinner or varied. For breakfast you only have 1 cup of coffee or teas of different flavors. That is what intermittent fasting is all about "Coffee, only on an empty stomach".

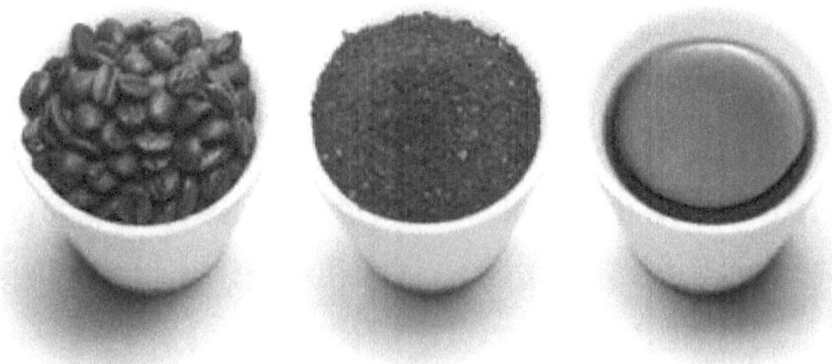

Chapter VII

Foods you should buy to lose weight
(Flexible)

In this chapter and the next one, I will tell you about all the types of foods you can eat for your diet. We in this book talk about (flexible feeding).

LIQUIDS

Liquids should not be counted in your calories, they do not satisfy, but if I recommend the liquids you should drink.

1. Water should always be in your life.

2. if you like soda and have a sweet appetite you can have soda (no calories). You have no restrictions, but I recommend these:
Coca Cola Zero, Sprite Zero, Fanta Zero, sugar free soft drinks.

It's funny because people complain about sodas and drinks, but sometimes they don't think that chicken, meat, are full of chemicals and hormones. In addition to the hundreds of other things like cars that pollute the environment and people who smoke near you. You have the decision to drink soda, I am not forcing you!

Carbohydrates

I like to recommend foods that are often in the "cannot eat in the diet" taboo.

1. Brown rice or white rice. You can consume any type of rice as long as you do it in small portions. I recommend brown rice because it contains a lot of fiber and few carbohydrates.

2. Light beans --- Per 16gr serving of carbohydrates, 11 Grams of fiber and 8 gr of protein. They are low in fat.

3. Whole meal bread (choose a bread that has a lot of fiber and few carbohydrates per serving).

4. Tortillas omelette (susalia) --- have a lot of fiber, and only 6 grams of carbohydrates.

5. Banana — provides many minerals, vitamins. (It is important to consume many fruits and vegetables)

6. Puffed rice --- In caloric deficit they provide few calories and you can eat in large quantities.

7. Oatmeal Cookies - After exercising it is a delight if you are in caloric deficit.

8. Green Tea.

9.

Healthy Fats

1. Walnuts

2. Almonds

3. Avocados — 7 grams of fat 4 carbohydrates and 2 grams of protein.

4. Coconut oil

These provide a lot of fiber.
There are many foods that have a lot of fat like ice cream foods that are not nutritious.

Protein

It is necessary to consume protein during a diet,

1. Dried meat — Very high in protein.

2. Tuna — high in protein.

3. Chicken salads

4. Navy blue — tuna with 15 grams of protein.

5. Lean meat — has a lot of protein and little fat.

6. Chicken and fish

7. Egg white — 10 grams of protein.

Fruits and vegetables

1. Frozen mango

2. Banana

3. Strawberries — contribute few calories.

4. Red fruits are low in calories.

Dairy products

1. Light milk

2. Almond milk - recommended for lactose intolerant people.

3. Cheese - consume low-fat and high-protein cheese.

Seasonings

You can consume any type of seasoning as long as it is low in calories.

Bonus Meals

1. Coffee is very good to speed up metabolism and to quench hunger. I recommend coffee low in sugars.

2. Change oil --- Use low-calorie oils.

3. Pumpkin is a food that due to its low calorie and fat intake is recommended to be included in your recipes.

Don't restrict yourself

Include what you like so much if you are sweet or you like many salty foods.
Remember 7% nutritious meals and 25% of foods not as nutritious as ice cream, tamarinds, chocolates, cookies.

If you think that some products are bad and can cause hundreds of diseases I answer that many things are more harmful to health such as smoking and addictions.

Chapter VIII
Healthy nutrition

Healthy nutrition is very important for weight loss or if you want to lose weight by eating only nutritious foods. -- :

FRUITS AND VEGETABLES

1. Tomatoes — Ideal for making sauces.
2. Lemons — Vitamins and minerals.
3. Mangoes --- Sweets full of minerals.
4. Avocado — Good source of fat and protein.
5. Lettuce --- Ideal in caloric deficit.
6. Tangerine — Juicy and rich in nutrients.
7. Chia - Ideal for burning calories and satisfying hunger.
8. Grapefruits — Contain many necessary nutrients.
9. Bananas — Sources of Carbohydrates.

You can decide which healthy foods to buy as long as you check and investigate that it does not contain many calories such as tamarind or coconut.

MEATS AND CHICKENS

1. Ground beef

2. Chicken breasts.

3. Lean meats

4. Tuna — to vary chicken and meat. You can also opt for fish or sardines.

PASTA AND CARBOHYDRATES

1. Quinoa — To vary the diet

2. Almond milk — it's great for breakfast or for coffee.

3. Wheat pasta.

4. Whole meal flour - for bread.

OTHER FOODS

1. Coffee — ideal for accelerating metabolism and for intermittent fasting.

2. Peanut butter — high in protein and very healthy.

3. Eggs — with high protein.

4. Walnuts

5. The most important — give yourself your taste:

 Don't feel that you have to limit yourself — remember that 15 or 25% of daily foods can flexible. If you do not want it that way and you are used to eating healthy foods you can also do it.

Chapter IX
Intermittent fasting
This is gold!

Fasting is not new, it is an ancient religious practice that is to spend long periods without eating food. Bringing intermittent fasting is quite simple for people, remember it is only a technique to push calories to the next meal.

Adapt your fast to your lifestyle

"As long as you can" without having to limit yourself or starve. You can fast 5, 8, 12, 14, 15 hours as long as you moderate your fast.

Mostly I recommend fasting if you start with 10 hours and then progress until you get used to it.

Benefits of fasting
- **Body fat loss**
- **Weight loss**
- **Fight diabetes and hypertension**
- **Fight allergies**
- **Reduces food and appetite addiction**

- **Reduce addictions such as nicotine and alcohol**
- **Combat depression and insomnia**
- **Improves metabolism**

Fasting Technique --

Fasting adapts to some lifestyles, we are all different, here my fasting technique:

1. I don't have breakfast, I get up, I only drink coffee to satisfy myself and feel energized to go to work.
2. At 1 in the afternoon I make my first meal, in total it is 13 to 15 hours of fasting if my previous meal was at 9 or 10 of the previous day.
3. My last meal is at 9 or 10.

Intermittent fasting allows you to distribute your meal in a single daily meal so that you are satisfied and eat what you want in a meal.
Remember to graduate so that your body adapts and no matter what hours your fast lasts, the important thing is the calorie balance of what is consumed in a day with the calories burned or spent.

Types of fasting

1. You can change the fast at lunch or dinner, you can also fast at night and it is extremely good and is what some instructors do with their students without telling them that it is intermittent fasting. They practically tell you that you should not have dinner, but they do not tell you that it is the technique of intermittent fasting. So if your last meal was at 2 or 5 in the afternoon, you postpone your dinner for breakfast and eat well at breakfast or vice versa.

2. Fasting 12 hours — 12 hours of fasting, 12 hours of feeding:

3. 7am des-fasting — 3pm healthy food- 7pm dinner (healthy option with some tastes)

4. 16 hours of fasting --- 8 hours of food — 10 am breakfast - 2 or 3 pm lunch — 7 maximum 8 dinner.

Coffee — coffee helps alleviate hunger for fasting, you can drink mineral water or teas with chamomile. Remember do not go crazy with a schedule and do not restrict yourself too much if you do not endure the desire to eat, it is not that your fast is accurate.
It is not for all intermittent fasting, but it is a beneficial technique to eat well without restricting yourself.

You must not go hungry

The people I tell about intermittent fasting think they will go hungry. The reality is that the body adapts because it is very intelligent, once adapted the opposite effect is usually achieved: less hunger. In a recent study, a group intermittent fasting reported less hunger than the group that made more meals. When analyzing hormones such as ghrelin and leptin (right), they found that they were effectively lower in the fasting group, and also observed improvement in basal metabolism.

Transformation of Olvera (authorized permission) with intermittent fasting

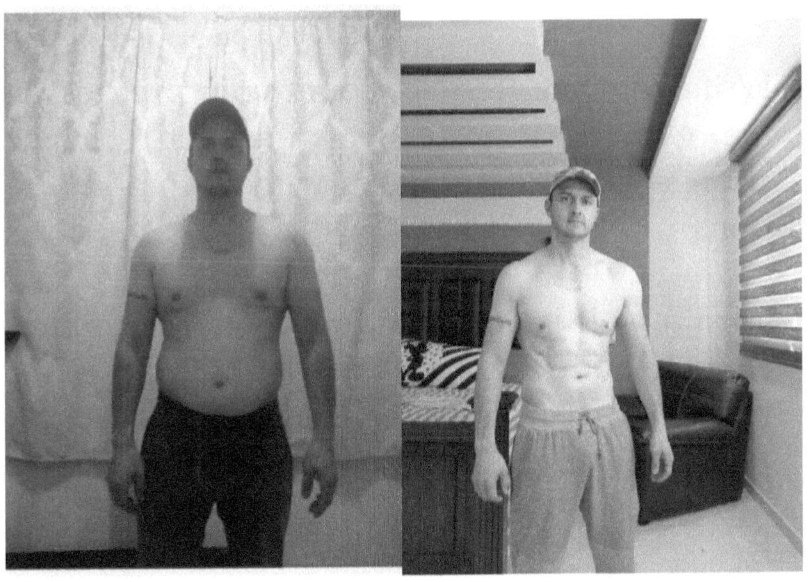

Chapter X

From obese to having a ripped abdomen

If you can go from obese to have a ripped abdomen like the one in the photo of the first pages.
Here 6 fundamental pillars in both men and women.

1. Flexible feeding --- The BEST diet is what you can do for the rest of your life and flexible is just that. If you're craving ice cream, have some ice cream! If you want a cookie, make a cookie!

2. Write your progress --- Count your progress in the gym and go progressing and become stronger in your abdomen with abdominals or irons.

3. Cardio --- It is very good to do cardio to burn enough calories, one of the best cardio is the HIT to burn calories after exercises.

4. Deficit — meals and calories. When you eat less and reduce your intake of what you eat daily, but do not forget to eat nutritious foods like all green spinach foods, broccoli, asparagus, green vegetables etc.

5. Patience --- Do not forget to have patience, just to read this book you have patience. Do not forget that the changes are not in 1 week or 2 weeks, this takes time because if you were in a bad diet and eating everything you wanted then you have to be patient to achieve your goals.

6. Do not train with weights! --- I have and I deeply believe that training weights is enough and better than cardio to lose weight. Remember that each person is different so do not follow the instructions of science and studies because I swear they are lies and distort the reality of fitness. You can do weights whether you are a woman or man. With the weights you burn fat, calories and build muscle. Do not be afraid to start carrying weight, you will not become like Arnold Schwarzenegger or if you are a woman you will become a bodybuilder. Bodybuilders use supplements and steroids to have a marked body.

Chapter XI
5 LIES OF THE FITNESS

5 lies that you believed about fitness and that is what prevents you from losing weight

1. Eating carbohydrates at night will accumulate as fat — there is nothing wrong with eating carbohydrates at night or in the day, you can eat them whenever you want, as long as you count how many calories you ate in the day and how many you burned.

2. Cardio more than 1 hour or repetitions of exercise greater than 2 hours — Exercise does not define whether you will lose weight or get ripped, what defines is your food, remember the food that enters and the calories you burn.

3. Avoid, bread, soda --- You should consume in moderation in small quantities or consume it in large quantities with your intermittent fasting, do not forget to consume fiber.

4. Genetics - no matter the genetics, you can have good or bad genetics and if you have a bad diet for more good or bad genetics you will gain or lose weight.

5. 5. Burn fat locally - You can't burn fat locally, but general fat! It is impossible to lower the fat where you want, even if you want it. If they tell you otherwise that with something you will eliminate fat they are lying to you. I don't say it but science does.

6. Believing in studies — Many times thousands of studies are distorted due to people's ignorance - I hear some say that they believe in studies of 5 or 6 people who went up or down or that the best diet is ketogenic, keto, or that the best way to get down is to take products from industries, it is not true!

I recommend you stop believing in studies but believe in the results of natural people and study people that worked for them and that — will apply to your lifestyle.

Chapter XII
Cardio to lose weight

In the gym I usually see a lot of people doing cardio to try to lose weight, but it is not the essential thing to lose weight, I usually see that they spend a whole night doing Cardio or even more than 2 hours in daily cardiovascular exercises. I even have friends who tell them not to do too much Cardio and ignore me for their stubbornness and I always see them the same.

Adapt

The body always adapts to everything you do; For example, it adapts in uncomfortable places or with people or friends, you adapt your income, your body also adapts in different situations.

In Cardio you have to be progressive! You cannot start with many hours of Cardio, you have to start with a few minutes and progress until your body adapts. Do not spend hours and hours! How many people have you seen that they continue doing cardio and see them the same? Remember you have to progress in your aerobic and strength exercises.

I cannot tell you how many hours you should do cardio but you have to do according to your resistance nor is it the way to lose weight.

My students have worked wonderfully less than 70 minutes of Cardio per week.

It is good for your health and has benefits to burn calories, but it is not the way to lose fat miraculously.

THE HIT ROUTINE

The high intensity Cardio is one of the best Cardio to burn calories in a short time. I do not say that he is the best, but he is one of the most people enjoy without spending hours and hours.

Hit House routine

Only 5 to 15 minutes, you can increase to 30 minutes if you have a treadmill or exercise bike. You can repeat it 3 times resting 1 minute between series and series.

1- 'Burpee' of 20 seconds.

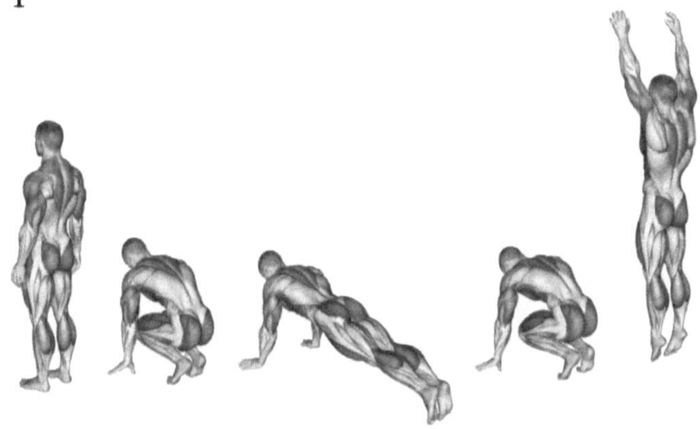

2- Knees up, 20 seconds.

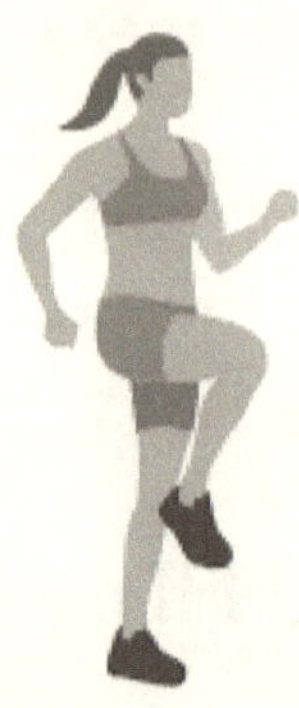

3- 'Jumping jack', 20 seconds.

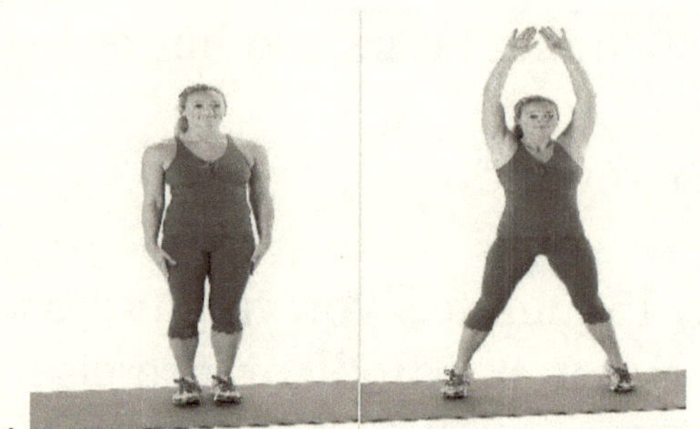

4- Squat (optional explosive squat), we will perform 20 seconds.

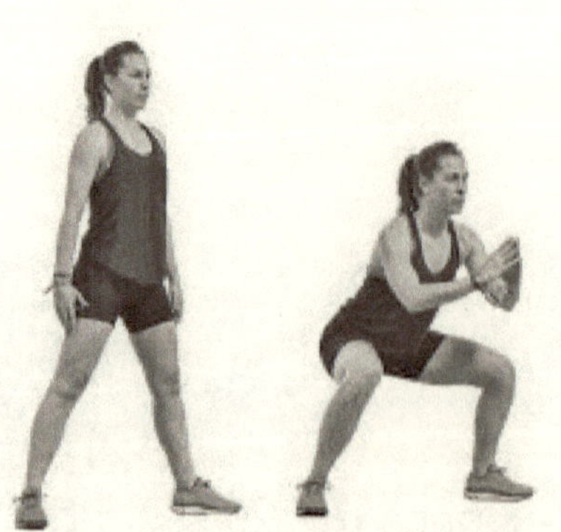

Bonus

1. Pushups

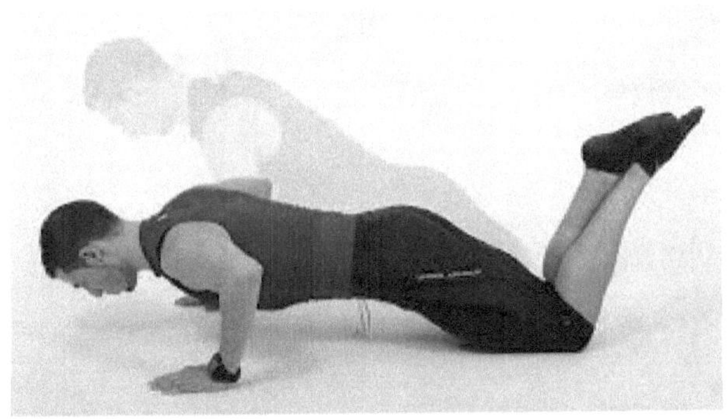

With progression

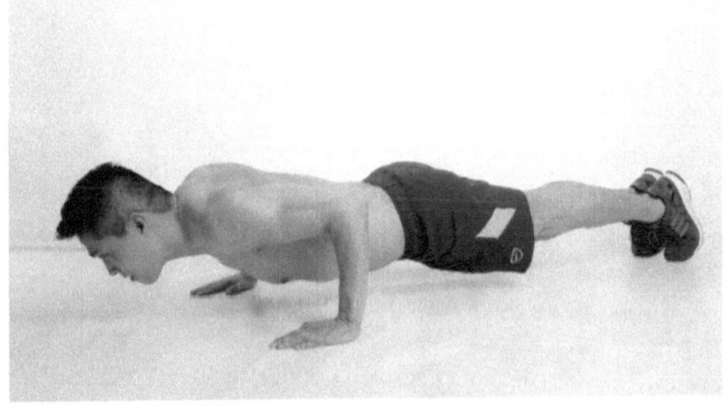

2. If you own these machines only 5 to 10 minutes

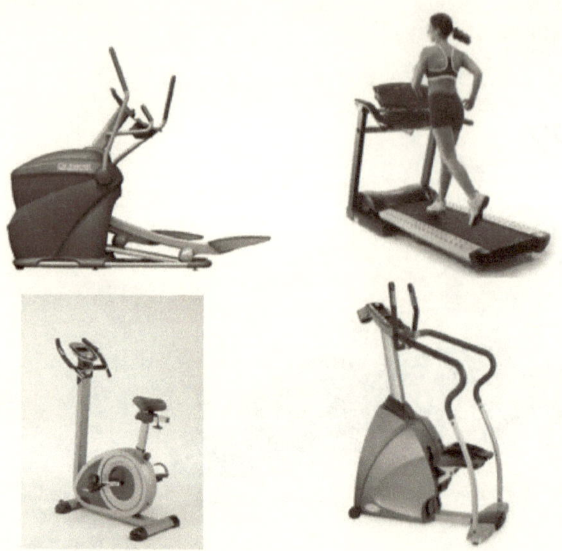

3. Dumbbell routine — triple 15 repetitions per exercise. 3 series.

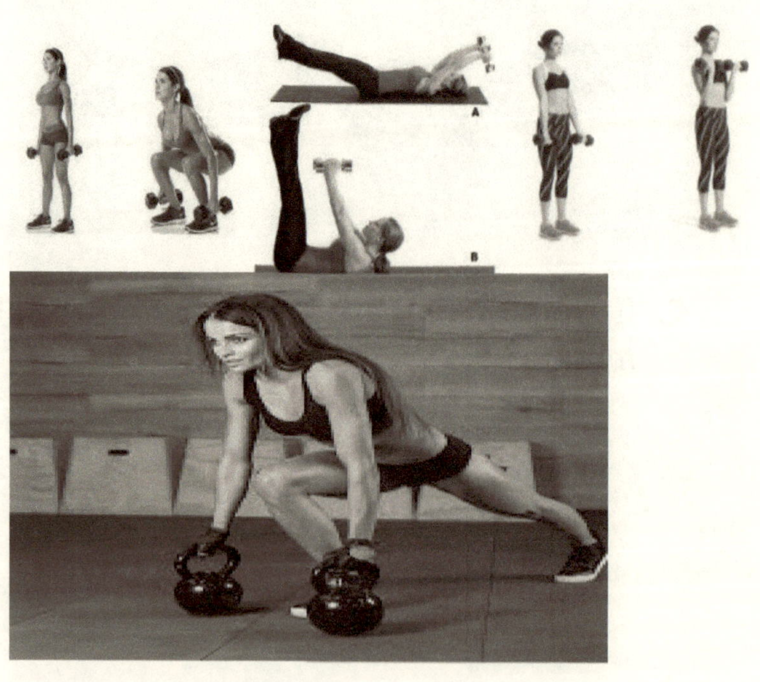

Weights are better than cardio

(Men and Women)

Women and men weight training. There is a myth that, in a few weeks of weight training, women will begin to see themselves with huge muscles and some men also avoid them because they don't like to have a good physique. Therefore many of them avoid doing weights at all costs, undergoing only cardiovascular work.

(Gaining muscle mass) is much more difficult for women than for men.

This does not mean that exercising with weights does not build muscle mass in women, but in less proportion than men due to what has been explained above.

But a woman with a good muscle mass will have a more active metabolism and therefore she will burn fat and lose weight faster. That's why toning with weights or dumbbells.

Prettier body ---

Here is differences between people who do weights and another who only trains without weights or does not exercise:

Without weights

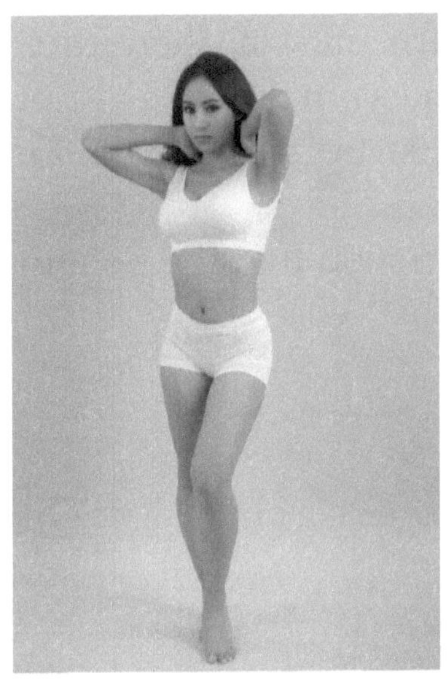

With weight and gym

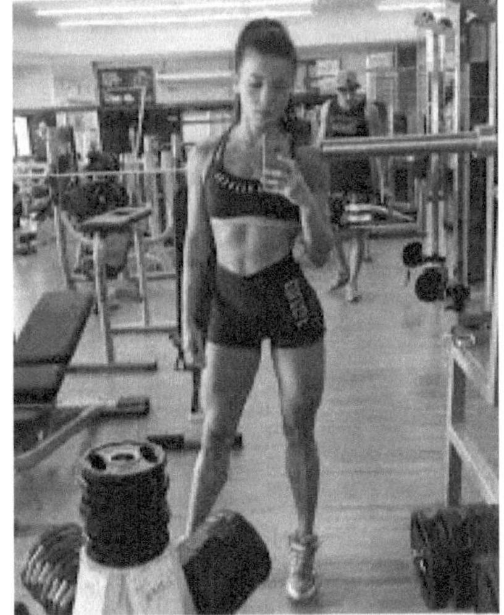

Then the food — with a good diet distributed in protein, carbohydrates and low fat dictates what will happen in your body.

Don't be afraid to carry weight — do squats, deadlifts, gain muscle, progress. When you lift weights you burn muscle, therefore, you burn more calories and tone your body. Do not expect to have the best physique by doing only Zumba or aerobic exercises.
As a man I assure you that the second photo is better.

Chapter XIII

Reduce waist and abdomen fat

We will work to eliminate fat from the waist --- Do not forget the philosophy of eating less than the calories you burn from fitness, it is not about counting but estimating and knowing that you should eat less every day.

Exercises:

1. Plank — very popular exercise.

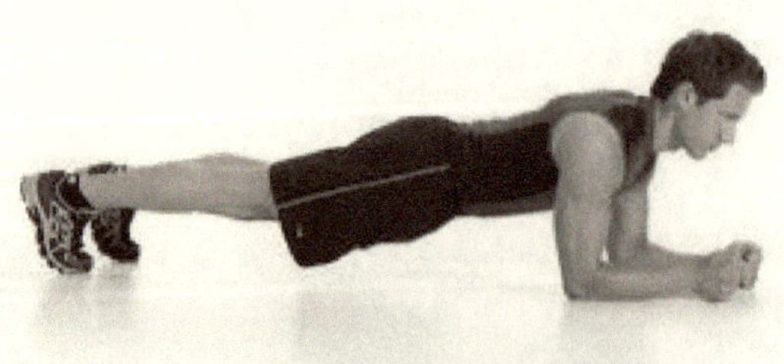

2. Mountain climbers.

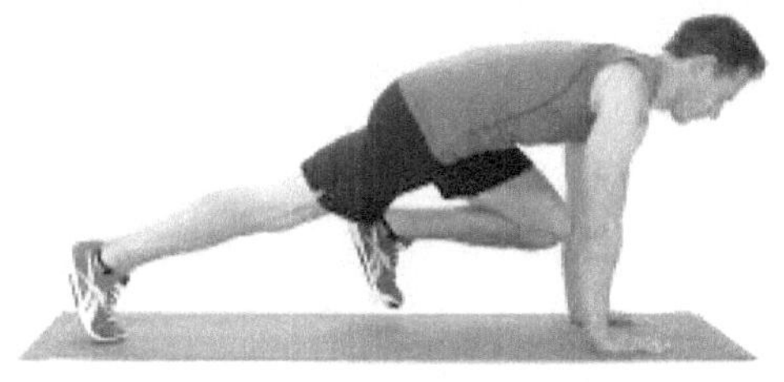

3. 3. Jump from side to side --

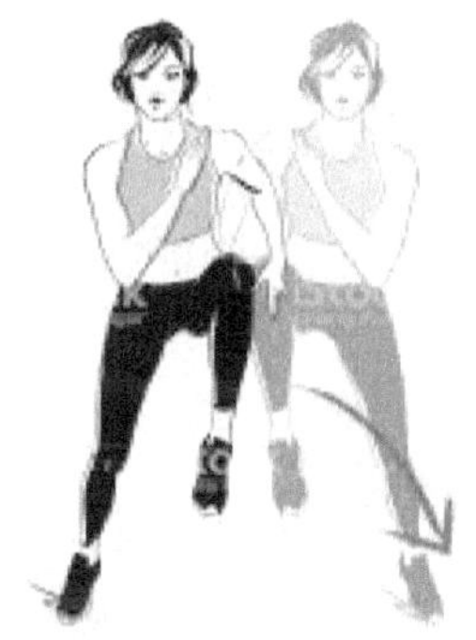

4. Optional jump –

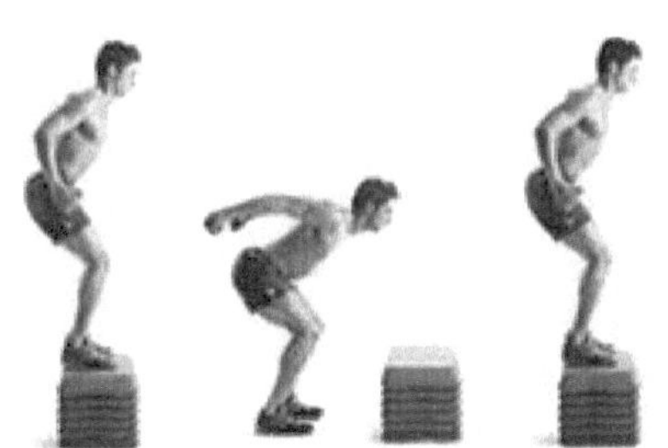

5. Buttocks, hip exercises —

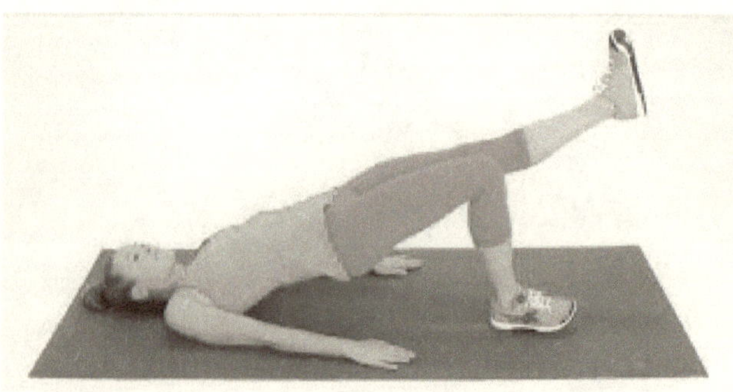

6. Hip and waist extension —

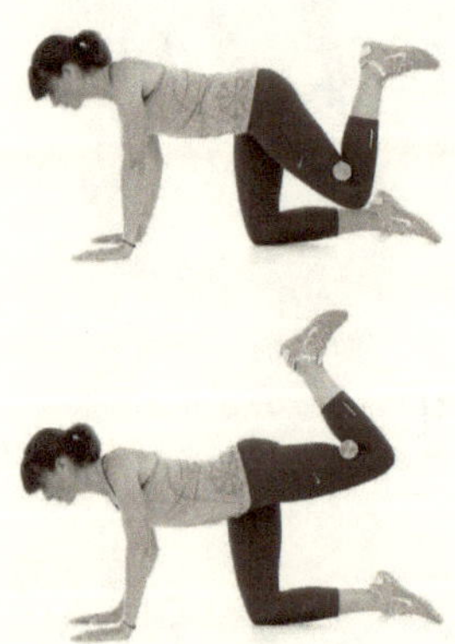

Remember to do it with the minutes you want as long as it is not too much, remember the work, commitment and emotional intelligence!

Chapter XIV
Caloric deficit

The caloric deficit is only a lack of calories in your day. Talking about a deficit is about reducing your daily maintenance calories. There is no exact number of what a person should consume in calories since each person is and does different activities.

If you consumed 3000 calories in the day and you remove 500 calories you will lose weight. Then if you consume 2600 calories for 2, 3 weeks your body will adapt to your new intake; Remember your body adapts as it is intelligent. Then you will have to increase your physical activity, walk more, and exercise to continue losing weight.

Remember that not only is the caloric deficit, but it must be a correct distribution of macronutrients in proteins, fats and carbohydrates.
Not only must you count calories, do not make the mistake of not only counting calories and eating only fat and scrap, but also counting macronutrients that are necessary.

In the vitality of the body it is necessary that you have a diet full of vitamins, fruits, vegetables, minerals, proteins, fibers.

Little by Little

Remember that you should decrease your caloric intake little by little. You cannot lose 1000 or 2000 calories overnight to your caloric intake without carbohydrates, or proteins because you most likely lose muscle, body shape, energy or you may fall into the rebound effect.

Caloric impact

Remember not to feel restricted from eating some foods. The diet or flexible diet gives importance to macronutrients; Remember and you should know that the body has no sensors to know if 150 gr of fries is the same as a piece or dish of chicken with cheese or ham. For the body they are the same calories, obviously the chicken with ham has and is more nutritious, but for the body regarding the calories it is the same; that is why you should not feel guilty of consuming in small quantities some foods that you like most.

Remember the most important thing that everything takes time. Thankyou

Chapter XV

Counting, estimating macros is important for weight loss

There are many people who do not know how to count macronutrients, they think it is difficult or that you have to take your balance every night or every day. But you must understand that it is only adding, what we were taught in elementary school. I will summarize:

Everything is based on proteins, carbohydrates and fats.

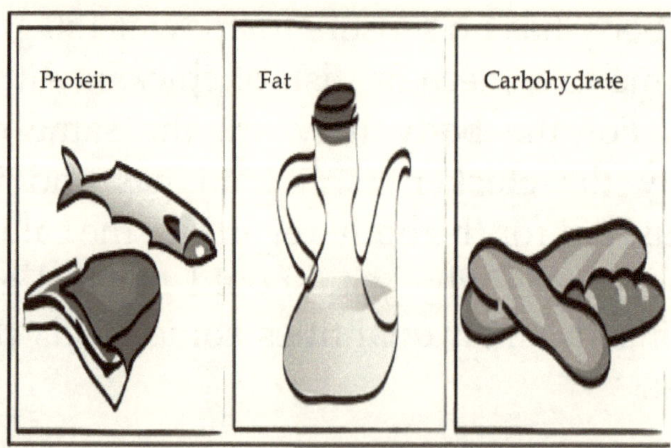

Remember that any food you eat has proteins, carbohydrates and fats (all) obviously some foods have 0 grams of fat or 0 grams of protein or 0 grams of carbohydrates.

There is no exact amount of what a person should consume in carbohydrates, proteins and fats, why? Because each person is different!

We will see some examples of how to distribute macronutrients, just an example does not mean that you should consume the same for your body. We will only give an example---.

140 gr of protein.	230 gr of carbohydrate.	45 gr of fat.

We'll start with protein --- Look for the best foods like chicken, tuna, fish, salmon, egg white, protein milk, protein powders (not necessary), peanuts, etc. These foods are the most abundant in protein, they are not the only ones.

150 GRAMS OF TUNA OR CHICKEN IS NOT THE SAME AS 150 GRAMS OF PROTEINS.

Remember that it is not the same weight as the nutritious of a product. Remember that 100 grams of chicken have 25 grams of protein.

Carbohydrates --- People complain about consuming more than 200 grams of carbohydrates. Look most products are full of carbohydrates; they are fruits, vegetables, rice, legumes, tortillas, potatoes, beans, cereals. It should not abound in carbohydrates, but remember the theory of 70% and 30%.

Fats --- These are cheeses, avocado or avocado, dairy (dairy products have proteins, but at the same time they have fats) almond milk and others.
Processed foods are full of fats. I recommend that your fats be from nutritious foods.

MACROS PER DAY

I always recommend using **MyFitnessPal or GOOGLE that has the answer to everything.** To count macros or estimate them if you feel lazy to count for yourself.

This is very simple math, just add and subtract. I will give you an example of mine:

Requirements

140 gr protein
230 gr of carbohydrates
45 gr of fat

It's 7 in the afternoon and I've consumed 90 grams of protein, 200 grams of carbohydrates and 35 grams of fat. Then I'm missing--:

50 gr of protein
40 gr of carbohydrates
10 gr of fat

Knowing what I'm missing, I try to fill the necessary nutrients with good food, such as --- chicken that contains 25 grams of protein per 100 grams. Then I consume 200 grams of chicken that helps me cover the necessary proteins and grams of fat because the chicken contains 10 grams of fat per 100 grams of chicken portion.
If I lacked 40 grams of carbohydrates you can eat everything green like vegetables, green foods to fill 40 grams of carbohydrates. Remember that you can consume some foods such as light beans, or consume it with normal or light rice.
If you have food or nutrients like carbohydrates, fill them with strawberries or cover your macros at the end of the day.

Mostly in the day I enjoy the food and leave the macronutrients and the strict diet for the night. ("Or you can do it the other way around")

Why should I estimate macros?

The only thing that matters in diets is to comply with macros. Diets that demand or restrict you in carbohydrates or fats end up failing losing muscle, energy and the rebound effect, science says.

Feel free to eat the foods you like most like breads, avocados, peanut butter or avocado, I also recommend using light oil without calories.

I don't know the macros or the nutritional value of restaurant meals, or event meals?

Remember to estimate macros in food if you don't know the nutritional value. In my **MyFitnessPal** there are plenty of event foods or fast foods that contain their nutritional value.

They are not exact results, but they are estimates. But I recommend sometimes in some processed foods increase from 30 to 100 calories. Exceeding calories in a certain time will make a long-term difference.

Don't restrict yourself

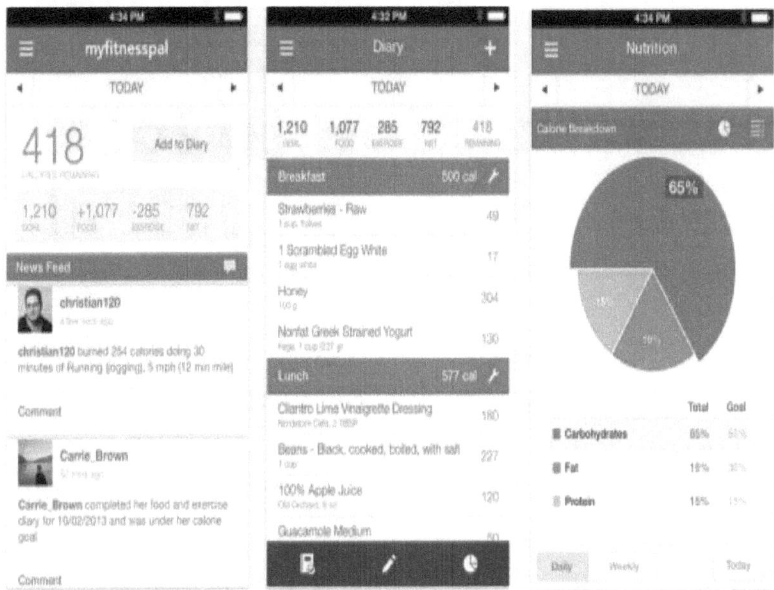

You should not take your weight to each place or tell people that you cannot eat rice or cannot eat such foods because you are on a diet. Do not kill yourself by weighing a fish or a meal or an ice cream.

Thanks for your reading.

Macros and customization to lose weight in MyFitnessPal

Each person is different therefore I cannot tell you the exact amount of calories or nutrients that you should consume for the reason that each person is different, weighs different, has a different age, eats different, measures different, has different jobs or routines.

But **MyFitnessPal** will get you an estimate of the calories and nutrients you should consume.

Create a profile in MyFitnessPal App

Register -> Register with email or Facebook -> Answer the questions -> ready

Set your macro or calorie goal

- Tap on Goals

- Scroll to nutrition and tap "Calories, carbohydrates, proteins and fats."

- Then adjust each macro with your desired target.

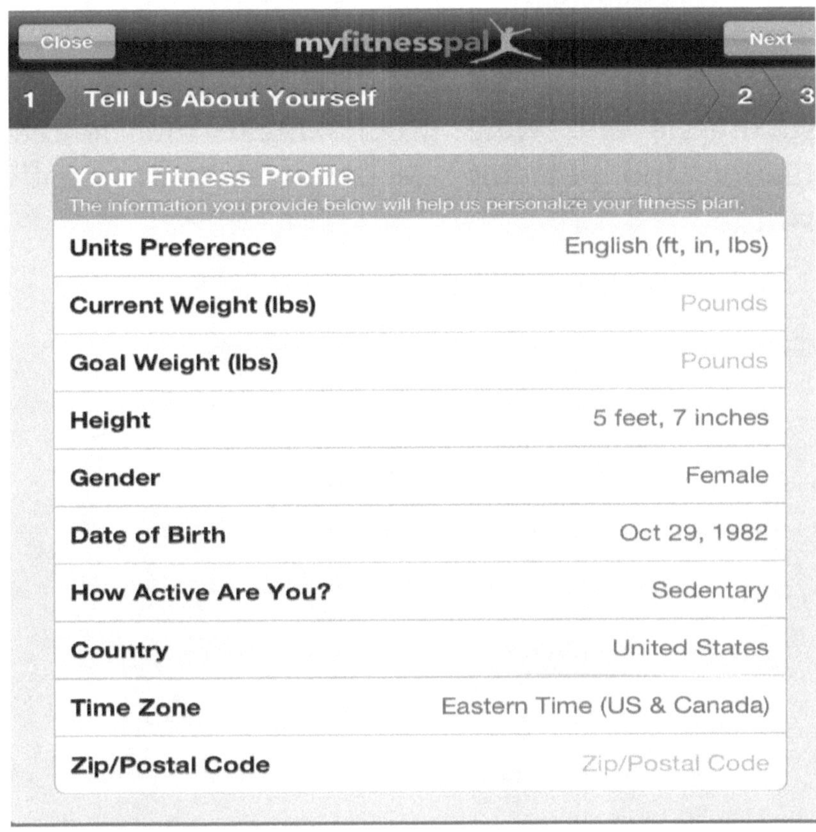

Remember to enter the correct data to have greater perfection in the calculation of the application metabolism.

as you begin to lose weight, your metabolism will begin to decrease too, that is, it will adapt; Eventually you will reach a point where you will not lose fat or weight at the same rate (or you will not lose anything) will stagnate and then you will have to create a new deficit and increase progression in strength, and cardiovascular exercises.

The metabolism will always adapt because you don't want to lose fat. It is advisable to lose 0.5 to 1% of your body weight per week and it is optimal not to lose muscle and water to maximize muscle mass retention and not stagnate or lower with negative results.

Chapter XVI
Calorie cycle per week.

The most important thing to have the best physique and succeed in your weight loss plan is adherence. In the pyramid of Erick Helms it is very clear:

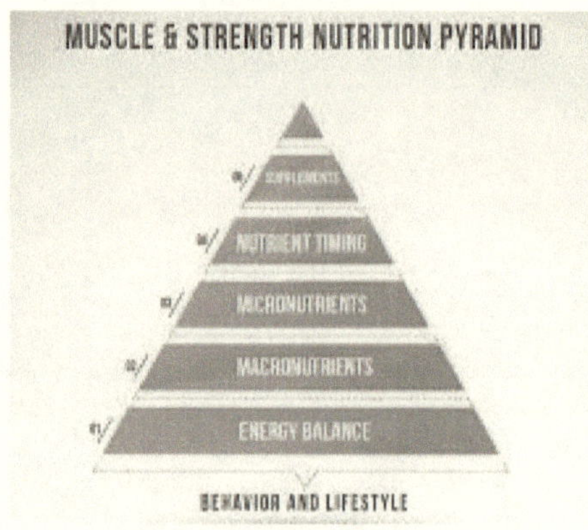

How does the adhesion phase work? - Works with macronutrients and calories.

Secret of the weekly macros

From now on I ask you to meet or do weekly phases of matching macronutrients in your days in the week. These examples are to avoid eating, going out, enjoying with your friends or partner, so you stop avoiding eating what you like most on some days of the week without having to limit yourself or restrict yourself.

We see 3 scenarios of matching macronutrients

1. Example for a woman

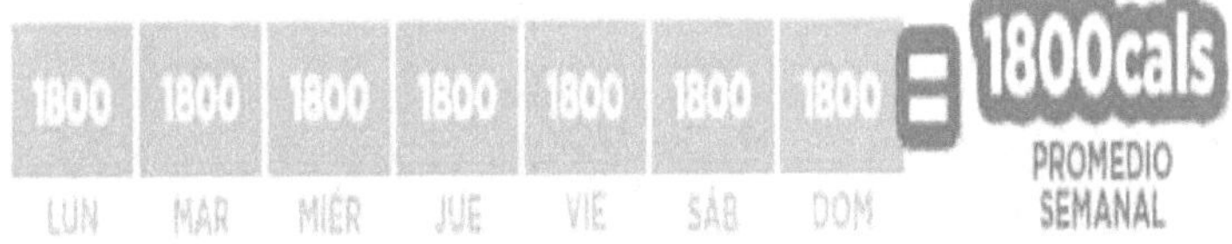

1800 calories per day, so your weekly average is 1800 average calories weekly.

2. Example of some people who eat more on training days.

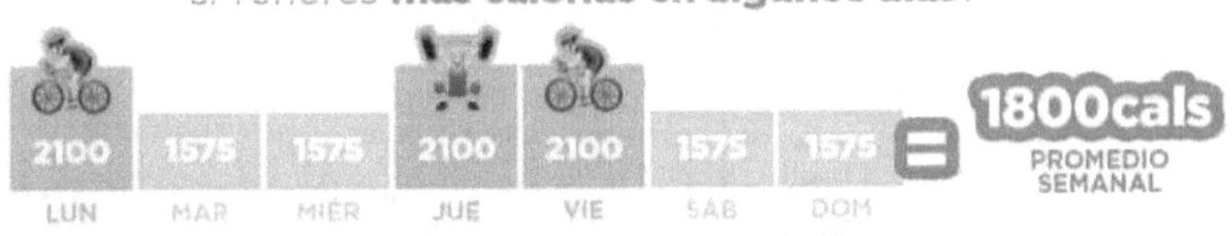

Adding the days that eat more in the days of divided training gives 1800 calories.

3. People who have couples or some events, then enjoy food on Fridays and Saturdays.

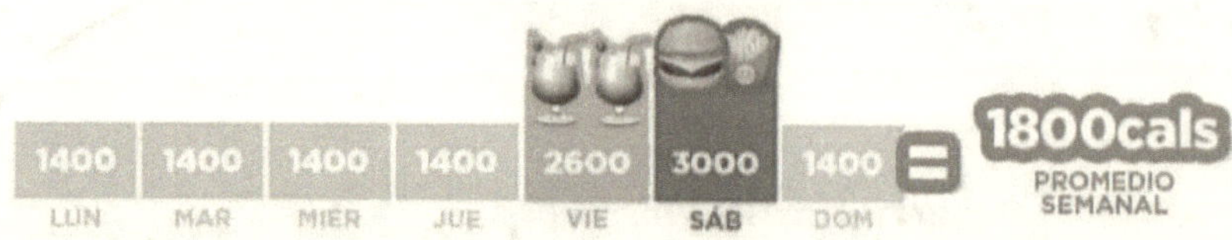

It is about eating 1400 calories during the week and on weekends you can eat with your friends, party, social events and enjoy adherence without having to say the typical word ("I'm on a diet").

You have the decision to choose between the 3 stages of macros.

How to overcome the days of low calories?

With intermittent fasting you will solve the days of caloric deficit or eat healthy during the week.

Remember the most important thing that-- it all takes time.

Thank you

Chapter XVII
Lose fat and not muscle

In this chapter we will talk about 2 different concepts.

It is not the same size as muscle. —Many people tell them that they should make a caloric deficit because they think that when they grow up they look good.

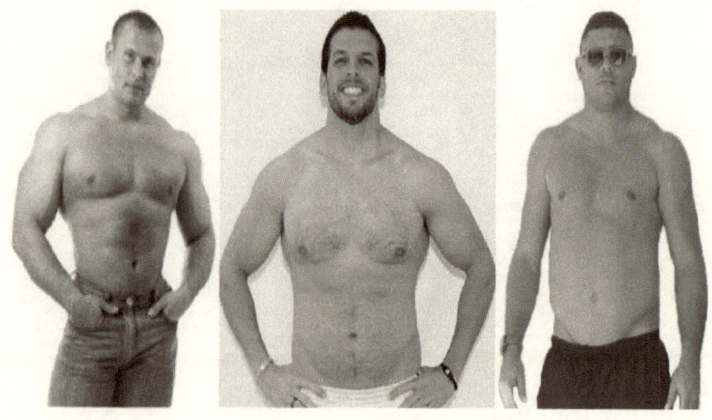

How many people have you seen that appear to be large, but do not have muscle, or notice your abs? --- The best thing I recommend to these mostly endomorphic people is to be in caloric deficit.

Catabolism --- Catabolism is a myth or what people are afraid of. It is impossible to catabolize with high body fat, because the body always uses fat to take energy in the caloric deficit.
If you are not like that then it is impossible to catabolize

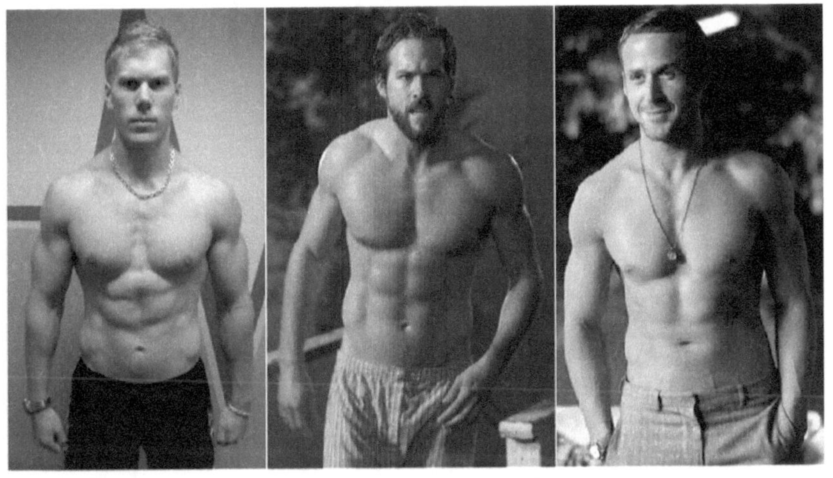

I swear I have asked several people which one is better and they tell me that the last image is 10 times better than being big without muscle.

But you have the last decision whether to get big or get a good physique with some abdomen pictures. At that time you see your abs, I recommend you take care of yourself and take care of your necessary protein consumption.

Chapter XVIII
You don't lose weight? (Accelerate your metabolism)

There are lots of tips to speed up metabolisms such as vinegars or many people use girdles or seek to find the only secret to speed it up. I give you 3 tips to speed up the metabolism.

1.   Build muscle mass --- As you build muscle mass demands muscle mass and energy to your body. The more muscle or mass your body will demand more energy. Remember that while you lose weight you should try to eat well and exercise to gain muscle.

2.   Spend more energy --- This advice is one of the best, it's about moving more, spending more energy on doing things, climbing the stairs, having sex, going for a run. The metabolism is composed of physical energy activity.

3.   Coffee --- Coffee is extraordinary and can help you speed up your metabolism. Remember that you should not abuse coffee because it has a long-term consequence. But it's very good because it helps burn fat and satisfy hunger.

Remember that --- **everything in excess is bad**

Don't spend your money

There are many products that often sell you their brand and make you believe that they will help you. Products such as vinegar or lemons to accelerate metabolism, pills to accelerate metabolism, Herbalife products, remember that decreasing fat is a consequence of caloric deficit.

Chapter XIXSupplements?

(Herbalife, Vivri, Omnilife, detox,)

There are many brands that "sell you miraculous products" to lose weight, supplements, pills, creams for the abdomen, belts that make you believe that you will effectively lose weight. --- The smoothies of these companies, although they are not harmful to health and may have some benefits, I think you do not need to spend too much money to those companies.

Rich Industries ---

These industries, although they help people is a very rich industry to sell brand and sometimes exaggerate to sell their products. It is also not bad that you buy them, but it is not necessary that you buy it or fall in ignorance with all due respect.

Reality

One day I heard an advertisement for a product of a company in which he offered his "miraculous product", it said this:
A: (Take our products 2 times a day, eat only one meal a day and you will lose weight easily.)

Clearly you will lose weight by only eating a daily meal if that meal has less than 500 calories. In what will end your body is indeed rebound or other problems caused by the abrupt change of calories.

Herbalife Challenge

One day a girl from the gym told me that she had lost weight thanks to Herbalife and was very grateful for the products so we started this conversation:

Q: "Hello Leonardo, I tell you that I have lost a lot of weight thanks to the products of this company ..."
A: "How good I am very happy, but tell me what do you eat per day?"

Q: "As a very light meal, I take my products on an empty stomach and before bed. I take my products 2 times a day and only light lunch"

A: "Look friend, I tell you that you don't lose weight because of the products, but because you eat low calories in your body"

You do not lose weight because of the products, but for the caloric deficit remember that.

You can continue to buy the products or not, but I recommend you and tell you that they are not necessary. Instead of spending and spending in the industries, it is best to spend on your change of healthy eating, to train other sports or to enter the gym.

What I recommend are vitamin products, omega 3 and natural foods such as fruits, vegetables and meet your necessary nutrients such as proteins, legumes, fibers and carbohydrates.

Chapter XX

I am Endomorph and Mesomorph how should I lose weight?

Many people asked me how to train if they were ectomorphs, mesomorphs, endomorphs, ectomorphs with mesomorph's touches, if they had poor genetics from their parents or a combination of the 3 body types. ---

I hear many times that they tell me —
A: Look, I eat small amounts and I don't lose weight, I think it's my genetics,

Or sometimes I hear some say —
A: what I eat I transform it into fat

And others ---
A: I eat a lot and I don't gain muscle mass
In fact, there are people whose fat deposits go to the waist, legs or face or in different parts, but it is no excuse to blame genetics for being endomorphic or mesomorph.

My thought is that we must all train and find the same way to lose weight --- If you made a deficit you will lose weight, if you made a surplus you will gain weight even if you are Martian or from another planet. Remember to distribute the necessary nutrients in your caloric diet whether deficit or caloric surplus

Remember to be patient because everyone wants to lose weight in a short time, on days in less than a month or with other formulas, but unfortunately it is difficult or worse it is still not recommended.

It is not magic to lose weight, but I assure you that, if you have a goal, training and feeding plan I assure you that you will lose weight in record time

Chapter XXI
Carbohydrates are your allies

The main element to lead a lifestyle and gain muscles including the abdomen are carbohydrates

If you continue with the diets to reduce carbohydrates to define you cannot get ripped or lose weight. Remember that your body adapts to carbohydrates and if you don't give it carbohydrates it won't be able to rip you because you won't have energy in your daily activities.

Carbohydrates are not to blame for you to gain weight or flour or bread if you reduce carbohydrates you will remain the same. With 130 grams of carbohydrates you will feel low energy while being overweight.

Carbohydrate myth

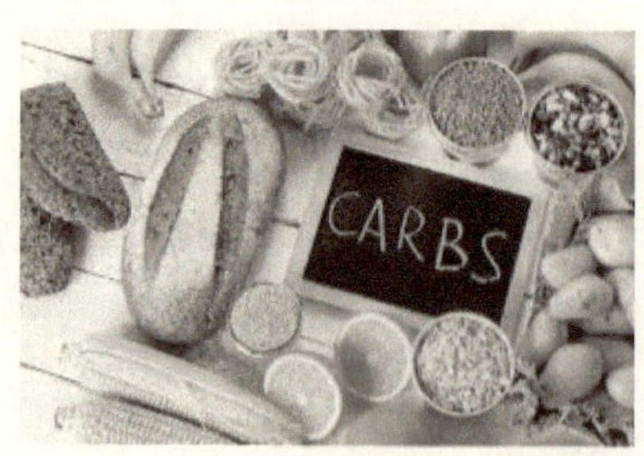

There are no bad foods that make you fat or that give diabetes or poisons. Everything in excess is bad because health is paramount, but, there should not be a total restriction of food and call them food poisons because they are simply defenders of "-healthy food", there are no harmful foods but with more nutrients than others.

You have the decision to continue eating vegetables, chicken with salad at the cinema with your partner with your Tupper, or with your bowl of vegetable food at events and be a victim of discomfort among friends and acquaintances.

But to those who really want to live a happy, healthy and unrestricted life, I recommend you continue with flexible eating.

Chapter XXII

YOUR SOCIAL LIFE IS MORE IMPORTANT DO NOT RESTRICT OR LIMIT YOURSELF!

Satanic people or restrict you to brands or label products as good or bad.

How many people have you heard say: --- you can't eat refined carbohydrates !, you can't have half a glass of soda, you can't eat 100 grams of ice cream once a week, you can't eat chocolate, you can't eat bread, no you can eat red or white meat, you cannot drink wine, you are mesomorphs with endomorphic touches therefore you cannot eat pasta or breads, you cannot eat tunas, you cannot eat or drink any Starbucks drink or any restaurant chain, you cannot drink milk at night, you cannot eat or drink any carbohydrates at night, you cannot drink dairy at any time of the day, if you eat this you will die in 3 days, or if you eat this you will die slowly and gain weight according to studies in the university of the united states:

That are nothing but lies because there is a saying —
"If a study says it is likely to be a lie".

Those people who forbid food or criticize food or worse still forbid you from eating meals or some foods as mentioned above are the same people who go with their partners or friends on Sundays and Saturdays to special events, cinemas, plazas, shopping centers , travel and eat everything they want. They are the same people who in their events drink wines and drink alcohol non-stop on special days. They are the same people who preach healthy food and cannot contain themselves and lie to themselves.

I deeply believe that you should lead a healthy life also with fruits, vegetables, vitamins, minerals, fibers and good proteins in your daily macronutrients. But that you also give yourself 30% of consuming your cravings or foods that you like the most.

The moment you restrict yourself or someone limits you, - then, you want it more ... do you remember that as a child your parents always restricted you something and you wanted to do it more?

This happens in life because we are designed to break the limits, so it is good to lead a healthy life with some foods that you like without having to restrict yourself. If you wish well, you can also lead a healthy life with restrictions, but I assure you that it will be harder for you to cope.

Chapter XXIII

Problems (stress, cellulite, excess skin and diseases)

Many people have problems when losing weight or have trouble accepting their reality. Do you prefer a lie, or a truth, even if it hurts? A lie is just self-deception. A pretext not to move forward, not to realize reality and hide so as not to face something that, however uncomfortable, will show you how to be a better person.

If you have some skin problems, gynecomastia, cellulite, excess skin after losing weight, it is best not to lie and go to the doctor to solve your problem. I give you 2 tips:

1.   Go to the doctor or a dermatologist-- That will reduce your excess.

2.   Ask for help --- if you have tried thousands of forms, creams and miraculous products do not continue doing the same and go to a true professional. Remember that everything has a solution.

Do not follow miraculous diets --

I constantly say that following miraculous diets is only a lie and they are not suitable for everyone. With those low carb diets or just eat fruits. It is not about losing 10 kilos in 2 weeks, if you do you will end up in rebound effect, with loss of water, muscle or problems of your organs due to lack of food.

Chapter XXIV

If you want to change things, don't always do the same

"Insanity is doing the same thing over and over again, but expecting different results."

- Albert Einstein

I love this phrase because it reflects a circumstance that occurs very frequently when it comes to losing weight. Faced with a certain problem there are people who repeat the same procedure over and over again, diets, creams, pills, shakes to lose weight. Maybe what they did before now is no longer useful because circumstances and science have evolved and the great truth that food is the main thing to lose weight has been uncovered.

Failure in various ways to lose weight repeatedly makes us begin to question ourselves "I am fat", "I have bad luck" ... We label ourselves negatively, lower our self-esteem and this makes us less effective.

As long as you keep doing the same, thinking the same, doing the same things, buying the same things and eating what you have been eating for a while, be sure that your results will always be the same, if you want a big change in your life you have to start doing big changes starting with food, exercise routine and in all aspects of your life, it's not easy, but it's worth it.

Chapter XXV
Motivation (Live your life be happy!)

Whenever the world turns its back on you, what you should do is turn your back on the world. Rudder.

Many times I have seen people who care about the thoughts of others and are afraid to set goals and achieve their dreams such as losing weight.

Don't despair

In just 2 months you will see natural changes in your body. The more you know about eating, ways to lose weight, the better your results. Stay updated with real information on ways to train better, nourish yourself better ... and when you see that little by little "in the mirror" you get results, you will not need more external motivations. There are a lot of training programs, ketos, ketogenic diets, etc., and if one of them doesn't work for you in a month, try another one until you find your dreams.

Also, today there are a wide variety of weight loss programs that can help you gain muscle mass, lose weight and fat. The important thing is not to give up and find a diet or weight loss program that suits your lifestyle, your way of being, your tastes, your social life and your time.
Get into a system that you know you can carry out in the long term.

Complicated

Who said it would be easy? If you don't like these tips, this is not for you. Remember that after the storm a beautiful sun rises.

Chapter XXVI

15 questions about losing weight (UNISEX)

1. Is food intake different for women?

Food for each individual is different, but flexible feeding can be done by any individual, whether male or female, because we are all human beings and we need macronutrients.

2. What should I have for breakfast?

It's a matter of taste, I recommend eating combinations of proteins, eggs, juices, fibers or something that gives you energy. Each person has resources, different tastes. Although you can practice intermittent fasting, (coffee) on an empty stomach and train.

3. Daily macronutrients I don't quite get there!

The changes do not come overnight, it is very important that you meet them daily. Although if you did not meet them you should reach weekly macros, that is, eat what you lack in protein the next day -

4. Train 7 days a week?

You should rest at least two to 3 days a week so as not to get tired of the routine.

5. Is it necessary to take supplements in powders?

It is only a supplement, I recommend natural foods since people have had bad effects after taking supplements.

6. Good and bad food?

According to science, the body does not know how to identify good and bad foods. It only absorbs proteins, carbohydrates, fats. It is good to have a healthy diet and if you eat foods called "bad" nothing will happen.

7. Lose fat and gain muscle at the same time

Losing fat = caloric deficit
Gain muscle and lose fat = make a slow deficit, which is slow but safe.

8. I did a diet and lost a lot of muscle, water and I have very flabby skin

The problem with diets is that you lose a lot of skin, water and muscles. I recommend you go to a doctor.

9. I want to gain muscle, I'm not too fat, what should I do?

The answer is in the mirror, if that happens to you I recommend you to make caloric deficit intelligently.

10. Should I lift weights if I am a woman?

It is very important to do weights whether you are male or female. With weights you burn more calories than doing cardio.

11.We all need different calories?

Yes, we all need different calories and macronutrients because we are different, we do different things, we weigh different, and we have different stature that is the reason.

12. The best food to lose weight?

Chia is the best food to lose weight due to its huge nutritional intake with low calories.

13. Should I continue with flexible feeding or do I continue with my old diet?

I advise you and I have told you in this book that you should be on a diet that you can take in the long term, ask yourself this --- Can I continue with this diet this year?

14. Where do I find its nutritional value of food?

On the internet, MyFitnessPal, and google.

15. Is it necessary to go to the gym to lose weight?

It is almost always better to go to the gym for machines and to try to burn more fat with weights and machines. Although you can do at home with your own weight.

Conclusion

Now you have learned how to lose weight in record time with natural benefits. Thank you for getting "lose weight without dieting" I hope this book is a tool to meet your goals. Soon the audiobook will be launched and volume II "lose weight and build muscle mass" Subscribe to our page to receive information about its release.

Before you go ....

Finally, if this book has helped you, I would appreciate your review in advance. This would help me grow and make more books to help people.

Find us on Facebook "Lose weight fast without dieting/ Leonardo Dominguez"